THE COMPREHENSIVE GUIDE
TO KEGEL EXERCISES

Boosting Pelvic Health, Confidence, and Intimacy

Adams .U. Morris

TABLE OF CONTENTS

CHAPTER 1

Introduction to Kegel Exercises

Welcome to the world of pelvic floor health and Kegel exercises. In this chapter, we'll embark on a journey to understand the fundamentals of Kegel exercises, which play a pivotal role in maintaining your pelvic floor's strength and overall well-being.

Understanding the Pelvic Floor Muscles:

To comprehend Kegel exercises, we first need to delve into the intricate structure of the pelvic floor muscles. These muscles form a hammock-like structure at the base of your pelvis, and their primary function is to support your pelvic organs, which include the bladder, uterus (in females), and rectum.

Imagine these muscles as a network of intertwined fibers, much like a woven basket. They cradle and hold your pelvic organs in place, preventing them from descending or causing uncomfortable conditions like pelvic organ prolapse. This supportive network is crucial for various bodily functions, such as controlling urination, bowel movements, and sexual activity.

Historical Background of Kegel Exercises:

Dr. Arnold Kegel, an American gynecologist, was the pioneer behind these exercises, which are aptly named after him. In the late 1940s, he developed these exercises as a non-invasive method to help women regain control of their pelvic floor muscles after childbirth. His work not only revolutionized postpartum care but also shed light on the importance of pelvic floor health for both women and men.

Kegel exercises have come a long way since their inception. They have evolved into a versatile set of exercises with applications beyond postpartum care. Today, they are recommended for a wide range of individuals, including those looking to improve their sexual health, manage urinary incontinence, and enhance core stability.

Benefits of Strong Pelvic Floor Muscles:

Now, let's explore why having strong pelvic floor muscles is essential for your overall well-being:

1. **Urinary and Bowel Control:** One of the primary functions of the pelvic floor is controlling the release of urine and stool. Strong pelvic floor muscles can prevent urinary incontinence (the involuntary loss of urine) and fecal incontinence (the inability to control bowel movements).

2. **Support for Pelvic Organs:** These muscles play a crucial role in supporting your pelvic organs. A weakened pelvic floor can lead to organ prolapse, where the bladder, uterus, or rectum drops from their normal position, causing discomfort and health issues.

3. **Enhanced Sexual Health:** For both men and women, strong pelvic floor muscles can contribute to better sexual health. They can lead to increased sexual satisfaction and may even

help with issues like erectile dysfunction and premature ejaculation in men.

4. **Core Stability:** Your pelvic floor is an integral part of your core. A strong core is essential for overall stability and posture, helping to prevent back pain and injuries.

5. **Pregnancy and Postpartum Recovery:** Expectant mothers can benefit from Kegel exercises to prepare for childbirth. After childbirth, these exercises can aid in the

recovery process and restore pelvic floor strength.

6. **Aging Gracefully:** As we age, our muscles tend to weaken. The pelvic floor is no exception. Regular Kegel exercises can help maintain muscle tone and prevent age-related issues like incontinence.

7. **Improved Quality of Life:** Ultimately, strong pelvic floor muscles can lead to a higher quality of life. They allow you to maintain control over bodily functions, enhance your self-confidence, and engage in

daily activities without fear of leakage or discomfort.

Now that we've established the importance of pelvic floor health and the potential benefits of Kegel exercises, you may be wondering how to get started. The journey to a healthier pelvic floor begins with understanding its anatomy, which we'll explore in detail in the next chapter. We'll learn about the different muscles that make up the pelvic floor and how they function to support your body and maintain its overall well-being.

CHAPTER 2

Anatomy of the Pelvic Floor

In this chapter, we'll take a deep dive into the intricate and vital anatomy of the pelvic floor. Understanding the structure and function of these muscles is crucial for anyone looking to embark on a journey to pelvic floor health through Kegel exercises.

Detailed Anatomy of the Pelvic Floor:

The pelvic floor is often compared to a sling or hammock that runs from the pubic bone at the front of the pelvis to the tailbone at the back. It consists of several layers of muscles, ligaments, and connective tissues. Let's break down its anatomy:

1. **Levator Ani Muscle Group:** This is the primary muscle group that forms the pelvic floor. It consists of the pubococcygeus, iliococcygeus, and puborectalis muscles. These muscles play a significant role in supporting the pelvic

organs, maintaining urinary and bowel continence, and contributing to sexual function.

2. **Coccygeus Muscle:** This muscle, also known as the ischiococcygeus, is located at the back of the pelvis and helps in supporting the coccyx (tailbone).

3. **Connective Tissues:** Collagen and elastin fibers make up the connective tissues in the pelvic floor, providing structural support. These tissues help maintain the elasticity and strength of the pelvic floor.

4. **Urogenital and Anal Sphincters:** The pelvic floor also houses the external sphincters, which are responsible for controlling the release of urine and stool. Strong pelvic floor muscles are essential for these sphincters to function correctly.

5. **Blood Vessels and Nerves:** A network of blood vessels and nerves supply the pelvic floor muscles, ensuring they receive adequate oxygen and nutrients and enabling proper muscle contractions.

Functions of the Pelvic Floor Muscles:

Now that we understand the anatomy, let's explore the essential functions of these muscles:

1. **Support for Pelvic Organs:** The primary role of the pelvic floor is to act as a support structure for the bladder, uterus (in females), and rectum. These organs rely on the pelvic floor's strength to stay in their proper positions.
2. **Urinary Control:** The pelvic floor muscles play a vital role in controlling the

release of urine. When these muscles contract, they help close off the urethra, preventing unwanted leakage.

3. **Bowel Control:** Similarly, the pelvic floor assists in maintaining control over bowel movements. Proper muscle function prevents fecal incontinence and ensures you can hold and release stool when needed.

4. **Sexual Function:** For both men and women, the pelvic floor is intimately connected to sexual function. Strong pelvic floor muscles can

enhance sexual pleasure, improve erectile function in men, and contribute to better orgasms in women.

5. **Core Stability:** The pelvic floor is an integral part of the core muscles, which help stabilize the spine and pelvis. A strong core, including the pelvic floor, is essential for good posture and preventing back pain.

6. **Childbirth Support:** In women, these muscles provide critical support during pregnancy and childbirth. A strong pelvic floor can help ease the

birthing process and aid in postpartum recovery.

7. **Maintaining Intra-abdominal Pressure:** The pelvic floor acts as a "floor" for the abdominal cavity. It helps regulate intra-abdominal pressure, especially during activities like lifting, sneezing, or coughing. A strong pelvic floor prevents issues like hernias and pelvic organ prolapse.

Common Issues Related to Pelvic Floor Weakness:

Understanding the pelvic floor's anatomy and functions also brings to light the potential problems that can arise when these muscles weaken. Some common issues related to pelvic floor weakness include:

1. **Urinary Incontinence:** Weakened pelvic floor muscles can lead to stress incontinence, where activities like coughing, laughing, or lifting cause unintentional urine leakage. It can also result in urge incontinence, characterized

by a sudden, strong urge to urinate.

2. **Fecal Incontinence:** Just as with urine, weakened pelvic floor muscles can lead to difficulty controlling bowel movements, resulting in fecal incontinence.

3. **Pelvic Organ Prolapse:** A weakened pelvic floor can fail to support pelvic organs properly, leading to conditions like uterine prolapse, cystocele (bladder prolapse), and rectocele (rectal prolapse).

4. **Sexual Dysfunction:** Pelvic floor issues can

contribute to sexual problems, including decreased sexual satisfaction and discomfort or pain during intercourse.

5. **Lower Back Pain:** Weak pelvic floor muscles can disrupt the stability of the core, leading to lower back pain and postural issues.

By gaining a thorough understanding of the pelvic floor's anatomy and functions, you're better equipped to appreciate the significance of maintaining its health. In the upcoming chapters, we'll delve deeper into Kegel exercises, how to perform them correctly, and their various applications in addressing pelvic floor-related concerns.

CHAPTER 3

Identifying Pelvic Floor Dysfunction

In this pivotal chapter, we delve into the signs, symptoms, and importance of diagnosing pelvic floor dysfunction. Awareness of these aspects is crucial because recognizing the presence of a problem is the first step toward effective treatment and management.

Signs and Symptoms of Pelvic Floor Dysfunction:

Pelvic floor dysfunction can manifest in a variety of ways, and its symptoms can differ from person to person. Being attuned to these signs is essential for early detection and intervention. Here are some common indicators:

1. **Urinary Incontinence:** The most recognizable sign of pelvic floor dysfunction, urinary incontinence involves unintentional urine leakage during activities like laughing, sneezing, or exercising. It can also manifest as a sudden,

uncontrollable urge to urinate.

2. **Fecal Incontinence:** This condition involves difficulty controlling bowel movements, resulting in accidental stool leakage. It can range from mild leakage to complete loss of bowel control.

3. **Pelvic Organ Prolapse:** Women may experience a feeling of pressure in the pelvic area or notice a bulge in the vagina, which could indicate pelvic organ prolapse. This condition occurs when the pelvic floor

fails to support organs like the bladder, uterus, or rectum, causing them to descend.

4. **Sexual Dysfunction:** For both men and women, pelvic floor dysfunction can lead to sexual problems. Men may encounter erectile dysfunction or premature ejaculation, while women may experience pain or discomfort during intercourse.

5. **Pelvic Pain:** Chronic pelvic pain can be a sign of pelvic floor dysfunction. This pain may be dull or sharp,

intermittent or constant, and can range from mild to severe.

6. **Incomplete Emptying of the Bladder or Bowels:** Difficulty in fully emptying the bladder or bowels can be a symptom of pelvic floor issues. You may feel the need to urinate or have a bowel movement frequently, even when there is little to pass.

7. **Back Pain:** Weak pelvic floor muscles can contribute to lower back pain, as they are a crucial part of your core's stability and support.

8. **Recurrent Urinary Tract Infections (UTIs):** Frequent UTIs may occur when the pelvic floor muscles do not provide proper support to the bladder, leading to incomplete emptying and bacterial buildup.

The Importance of Diagnosis and Assessment:

While it's crucial to recognize the signs and symptoms of pelvic floor dysfunction, obtaining a professional diagnosis is equally essential. Here's why:

1. **Tailored Treatment:** Proper diagnosis allows healthcare providers to tailor treatment plans to your specific condition. Not all pelvic floor issues are the same, and individualized care is essential for effective management.

2. **Ruling Out Other Conditions:** Many symptoms of pelvic floor dysfunction overlap with other medical conditions. A thorough assessment helps rule out other potential causes of your symptoms,

ensuring you receive the appropriate treatment.

3. **Preventing Progression:** Early diagnosis and intervention can prevent the progression of pelvic floor issues. Addressing these concerns promptly can improve your quality of life and prevent complications.

4. **Optimizing Recovery:** For those who have undergone childbirth, surgery, or other medical procedures that may impact the pelvic floor, an assessment can help optimize the recovery

process and identify any issues that need attention.

Seeking Professional Help for Pelvic Floor Issues:

If you experience any of the signs or symptoms mentioned earlier, it's crucial to seek professional guidance. Healthcare providers who specialize in pelvic floor health, such as urogynecologists, pelvic floor physical therapists, or urologists, can conduct a comprehensive assessment.

During your assessment, you can expect:

- **Medical History Review:** Your healthcare provider will ask about your medical history, including any surgeries, pregnancies, or relevant health issues.

- **Physical Examination:** A physical examination, including an internal pelvic exam, may be performed to assess the strength and function of your pelvic floor muscles.

- **Diagnostic Tests:** Depending on your symptoms, your provider may recommend additional tests, such as urodynamic testing to assess bladder function or imaging studies to evaluate pelvic organ position.

- **Discussion of Symptoms:** Open communication about your symptoms, their duration, and their impact on your life is vital. Be prepared to discuss these details with your healthcare provider.

Once your assessment is complete, your healthcare provider will work with you to develop a treatment plan tailored to your specific needs. This may include Kegel exercises, physical therapy, lifestyle modifications, medications, or, in some cases, surgical interventions.

Understanding the signs and symptoms of pelvic floor dysfunction and the importance of seeking professional help is the first step toward addressing and managing these issues effectively. In the upcoming chapters, we will explore how Kegel exercises can be an integral part of your journey to pelvic floor health.

CHAPTER 4

Basics of Kegel Exercises

In this chapter, we will delve into the fundamentals of Kegel exercises, providing a clear understanding of what they are, how to locate the pelvic floor muscles, the importance of proper technique, and setting realistic goals for your Kegel routine.

What Are Kegel Exercises?

Kegel exercises, also known as pelvic floor exercises, are a series of voluntary contractions and relaxations of the pelvic floor muscles. These exercises are named after Dr. Arnold Kegel, who introduced them in the 1940s as a way to strengthen these critical muscles.

Locating the Pelvic Floor Muscles:

Before diving into Kegel exercises, it's essential to know how to identify and isolate the pelvic floor muscles. These muscles are not visible, so finding them requires some mindfulness:

1. **Stop the Urine Flow:** While urinating, try to stop

the flow of urine mid-stream. The muscles you engage to do this are your pelvic floor muscles. However, this is only a practice method and should not be done regularly as a form of exercise.

2. **Imagine Stopping Gas:** Another way to identify these muscles is to envision preventing the release of gas. The muscles you contract to achieve this are part of your pelvic floor.

3. **Internal Sensation:** Alternatively, you can insert a clean finger into your

vagina (for women) or rectum (for men) and attempt to squeeze the muscles around your finger. You should feel a subtle tightening and lifting sensation.

Once you've located these muscles, you're ready to start your Kegel exercises.

Correct Posture and Breathing Techniques for Kegels:

Proper posture and breathing are crucial when performing Kegel exercises. Here's how to ensure you're doing them correctly:

1. **Posture:** Sit or stand up straight with your feet shoulder-width apart. Keep your shoulders relaxed and your chest lifted. Maintain a neutral spine position to avoid arching your back or tilting your pelvis forward or backward.

2. **Breathing:** Breathe naturally throughout the exercises. Avoid holding your breath. Inhale gently through your nose, and as you exhale, engage your

pelvic floor muscles, drawing them upward.

The Importance of Proper Technique:

Maintaining proper technique is essential for the effectiveness of Kegel exercises and to avoid potential issues:

1. **Avoid Overexertion:** Do not squeeze your pelvic floor muscles too hard. Instead, aim for a gentle contraction. Overexertion can lead to muscle fatigue and discomfort.

2. **Consistency is Key:**
Perform your Kegel exercises regularly. Like any form of exercise, consistency yields better results. You can start with a few sets a day and gradually increase the repetitions over time.

3. **Balanced Contraction and Relaxation:**
Remember that Kegel exercises involve both contraction and relaxation of the pelvic floor muscles. It's crucial to release the muscles completely between contractions.

4. **Patience and Persistence:** Results from Kegel exercises may not be immediate. It takes time to strengthen these muscles. Be patient and persistent in your practice.

Setting Realistic Goals:

When embarking on your Kegel exercise journey, it's essential to set realistic goals. Understand that the progress varies from person to person. Here's how to approach goal-setting:

1. **Know Your Baseline:** Start by assessing your

current pelvic floor strength. How long can you hold a contraction? How many repetitions can you do comfortably?

2. **Set Achievable Goals:** Begin with achievable goals. For example, if you can comfortably hold a contraction for five seconds, aim to increase it to ten seconds over a few weeks.

3. **Gradual Progression:** As you achieve your initial goals, gradually increase the duration of contractions and the number of repetitions. But remember, it's not a

race. Slow and steady progress is more sustainable.

4. **Regular Evaluation:** Periodically assess your progress and adjust your goals accordingly. This helps keep your motivation high and ensures you continue to challenge your pelvic floor muscles.

In this chapter, we've laid the foundation for your Kegel exercise practice by explaining what Kegels are, how to locate the pelvic floor muscles, the importance of proper technique, and setting realistic goals. In the chapters to come, we will explore in more detail how to design a personalized Kegel exercise routine, how to progress and intensify your workouts, and how to incorporate Kegels into your daily life effectively.

CHAPTER 5

The Kegel Exercise Routine

In this chapter, we will dive into the practical aspect of Kegel exercises. We will discuss how to design a personalized Kegel exercise routine, how to progress and intensify your workouts, and how to incorporate Kegels into your daily life effectively.

Designing a Personalized Kegel Exercise Routine:

A personalized Kegel exercise routine is essential because individual needs and strengths vary. Here's how to create a routine tailored to your specific requirements:

1. **Consult a Healthcare Provider:** If you have identified pelvic floor issues or are unsure where to begin, it's wise to consult a healthcare provider, such as a urogynecologist or pelvic floor physical therapist. They can assess your condition and provide guidance on the most appropriate exercises.

2. **Start with a Baseline Assessment:** Begin with a baseline assessment of your pelvic floor strength and endurance. This helps you gauge your starting point and track progress.

3. **Set Specific Goals:** Determine what you want to achieve with your Kegel exercises. Do you aim to improve bladder control, enhance sexual function, or alleviate pelvic pain? Your goals will shape your routine.

4. **Choose the Right Kegel Exercises:** Not all Kegel

exercises are the same. There are variations, including quick contractions, slow contractions, and sustained holds. Your healthcare provider can help you select the exercises that align with your goals.

5. **Establish a Routine:** Plan when and where you will perform your Kegel exercises. Consistency is key, so aim for a specific time each day to practice, such as after waking up or before going to bed.

6. **Warm-Up and Cool Down:** Like any exercise,

it's essential to warm up and cool down your pelvic floor muscles. You can do this by contracting and relaxing them gently for a few seconds before and after your main Kegel routine.

Progression and Intensity Levels:

As with any exercise regimen, it's crucial to progressively challenge your pelvic floor muscles to achieve results. Here's how to do it safely:

1. **Gradual Increases:** Start with a comfortable number

of repetitions and a duration that you can manage without straining. Over time, gradually increase the number of repetitions and the duration of contractions.

2. **Intensity Levels:** You can vary the intensity of your Kegel exercises. For instance, you can begin with gentle contractions and then progress to stronger ones as your muscles become more conditioned.

3. **Use Props:** Some individuals benefit from using props like vaginal weights or Kegel exercise

balls to add resistance and challenge to their workouts. Consult your healthcare provider before incorporating such props.

4. **Feedback Devices:** There are feedback devices available that can help you monitor your progress and ensure you are contracting and relaxing your pelvic floor muscles correctly.

5. **Consistent Evaluation:** Regularly assess your progress and adjust your routine accordingly. Your goals may evolve as you experience improvements in

pelvic floor strength and function.

Incorporating Kegels into Daily Life:

To maximize the benefits of Kegel exercises, it's essential to integrate them into your daily life seamlessly. Here's how to do it effectively:

1. **Reminders:** Set reminders on your phone or use cues like specific daily activities (e.g., brushing your teeth) to prompt your Kegel exercises.

2. **Scheduled Breaks:** If you have a sedentary job, take

short breaks to perform your exercises. This not only reinforces the habit but also helps prevent muscle fatigue and strain from prolonged sitting.

3. **Combine with Other Activities:** You can perform Kegel exercises during other activities, such as watching TV, reading, or waiting in line. No one will know you're doing them, and they can become a natural part of your daily routine.

4. **Partner Support:** Share your exercise goals with your partner. They can offer

encouragement and remind you to stay consistent.

5. **Mindfulness Practice:** Incorporate mindfulness techniques into your routine. This can help you stay focused during your exercises and enhance their effectiveness.

6. **Track Your Progress:** Maintain a journal or use a smartphone app to track your Kegel exercise sessions and record any changes in symptoms or strength.

Listening to Your Body:

While it's important to stick to your Kegel exercise routine, it's equally crucial to listen to your body. If you experience discomfort, pain, or any unusual symptoms during or after your exercises, consult your healthcare provider immediately. They can help you adjust your routine or identify any underlying issues that need attention.

In this chapter, we've covered the practical aspects of Kegel exercises. Designing a personalized routine, progressively challenging your muscles, and incorporating Kegels into your daily life are all essential steps in achieving the best results. In the chapters ahead, we'll explore how Kegel exercises can benefit specific populations, such as pregnant individuals, postpartum recovery, men's health, and aging adults.

CHAPTER 6

Kegels for Special Populations

In this chapter, we will explore how Kegel exercises can be tailored to meet the specific needs of various populations, including pregnant individuals, postpartum recovery, men's health, and aging adults. Each of these groups can benefit from Kegel exercises in unique ways, and understanding these applications is essential for effective pelvic floor health management.

Kegels During Pregnancy:

1. *Preparation for Childbirth:* Kegel exercises can be immensely beneficial during pregnancy. As the uterus expands and places increased pressure on the pelvic floor, these exercises can help prepare the muscles for the demands of labor and delivery. Strong pelvic floor muscles may enhance your ability to push during childbirth and promote quicker recovery afterward.

2. *Reducing Urinary Incontinence:* Pregnant

individuals often experience urinary incontinence due to the pressure on the bladder. Regular Kegel exercises can help strengthen the pelvic floor muscles and reduce the incidence of stress incontinence during pregnancy.

3. *Postpartum Recovery:* Continuing Kegel exercises postpartum can accelerate recovery. However, it's essential to consult with a healthcare provider before resuming exercises after childbirth, as the timing and approach may vary

depending on your individual circumstances.

Kegels for Postpartum Recovery:

1. *Restoring Pelvic Floor Strength:* After childbirth, the pelvic floor muscles can be stretched and weakened. Kegel exercises are a valuable tool in the postpartum recovery process, helping to restore strength and support to these muscles.

2. *Managing Pelvic Organ Prolapse:* Some individuals may experience pelvic organ

prolapse after childbirth, where the bladder, uterus, or rectum descends into the vaginal canal. Kegel exercises, when performed correctly and under professional guidance, can help alleviate symptoms and support the pelvic organs.

3. *Enhancing Sexual Health:* Postpartum women may also find that Kegel exercises contribute to improved sexual health, helping to alleviate any discomfort or changes in sexual function that may have occurred

during pregnancy and childbirth.

Kegels for Men's Health:

1. *Erectile Dysfunction (ED):* Kegel exercises are not exclusive to women; they can also benefit men. Some men experience erectile dysfunction due to weakened pelvic floor muscles. Kegel exercises can help improve blood flow to the pelvic region, potentially enhancing erectile function.

2. *Premature Ejaculation (PE):* Men who experience premature ejaculation may

find that Kegel exercises, specifically the ability to control and strengthen the pelvic floor muscles, can help increase ejaculatory control.

3. *Prostate Health:* For individuals dealing with prostate issues, such as prostatitis or post-prostatectomy, Kegel exercises can aid in maintaining urinary continence and supporting overall pelvic health.

Kegels for Aging Adults:

1. *Maintaining Continence:* As we age, the risk of urinary incontinence and fecal incontinence increases. Kegel exercises can be an effective tool in preventing and managing these issues, allowing older adults to maintain their independence and quality of life.

2. *Preventing Pelvic Organ Prolapse:* The risk of pelvic organ prolapse also rises with age. Regular Kegel exercises can help prevent or alleviate this condition, reducing discomfort and the

need for surgical intervention.

3. *Supporting Core Stability:* Aging adults can benefit from Kegel exercises as part of a broader strategy to maintain core stability, which is essential for balance, posture, and preventing falls.

Caution and Professional Guidance:

While Kegel exercises can be highly beneficial for these special populations, it's crucial to approach them with care and seek professional guidance when necessary. Every individual's situation is unique, and what works for one person may not work for another. Here are some key points to keep in mind:

- Consult with a healthcare provider, such as a urogynecologist, pelvic floor physical therapist, or urologist, before starting Kegel exercises, especially if you have specific medical conditions or concerns.
- Ensure that you are performing Kegel exercises correctly to avoid potential

issues like muscle overuse or fatigue.

- Be patient and realistic about your expectations. Progress may take time, especially if you are addressing long-standing issues.
- If you experience any discomfort, pain, or worsening of symptoms during or after Kegel exercises, consult your healthcare provider promptly.
- Consider incorporating other forms of exercise, such as core-strengthening exercises

and stretches, to complement your Kegel routine and promote overall pelvic health.

In this chapter, we've explored how Kegel exercises can be adapted to suit the needs of special populations, including pregnant individuals, those in postpartum recovery, men seeking improved sexual health, and aging adults. Understanding the unique benefits and considerations for each group empowers individuals to take control of their pelvic floor health and overall well-being. In the following chapters, we will delve into complementary exercises, dietary considerations, and mind-body techniques that can further enhance pelvic floor wellness.

CHAPTER 7

Beyond Kegel Exercises

In this chapter, we will explore additional strategies and practices that can complement Kegel exercises for holistic pelvic floor wellness. These include complementary exercises and stretches, dietary considerations, and mind-body techniques. Combining these approaches with Kegel exercises can contribute to comprehensive pelvic floor health.

Complementary Exercises and Stretches:

1. **Yoga:** Yoga can be a valuable addition to your pelvic floor health regimen. Certain yoga poses, such as Cat-Cow, Bridge, and Child's Pose, can help stretch and strengthen the pelvic floor muscles. Yoga also emphasizes deep breathing and mindfulness, which can enhance your overall awareness of your body, including the pelvic region.

2. **Pilates:** Pilates is another exercise modality that can

complement Kegel exercises. Many Pilates exercises focus on core strength, which includes the pelvic floor. Movements that emphasize core stability can help improve pelvic floor support.

3. **Squats:** Squats are excellent for strengthening the muscles of the lower body, including the pelvic floor. They engage multiple muscle groups simultaneously, promoting overall strength and stability. However, it's essential to perform squats

with proper form to avoid straining the pelvic floor.

4. **Hip Flexor Stretches:** Stretching the hip flexors can relieve tension in the pelvic region. Tight hip flexors can contribute to pelvic floor dysfunction, so incorporating hip flexor stretches into your routine can be beneficial.

5. **Pelvic Tilts:** Pelvic tilts involve gently rocking your pelvis forward and backward while lying on your back. This exercise can help improve pelvic mobility and alignment.

6. **Bridges:** Bridges are effective for both pelvic floor strengthening and lower back pain relief. They target the glutes and lower back muscles while engaging the pelvic floor.

7. **Core-Strengthening Exercises:** Exercises that target the core, such as planks and leg raises, indirectly engage the pelvic floor muscles. A strong core provides better support for the pelvic organs and can reduce the risk of pelvic floor issues.

Dietary Considerations:

1. **Hydration:** Proper hydration is crucial for overall health, including the health of the pelvic floor. Staying hydrated helps maintain optimal urinary function and can reduce the risk of urinary tract infections (UTIs).

2. **Fiber-Rich Diet:** Constipation and straining during bowel movements can strain the pelvic floor. A diet rich in fiber can promote regular and comfortable bowel

movements, reducing the risk of pelvic floor dysfunction.

3. **Limit Caffeine and Alcohol:** Caffeine and alcohol can irritate the bladder and lead to increased urgency and frequency of urination. Reducing your intake of these substances may help manage urinary symptoms.

4. **Bladder-Friendly Foods:** Some individuals with overactive bladder or urinary urgency find relief by avoiding certain bladder-irritating foods, such as

spicy foods, citrus fruits, and carbonated beverages.

5. **Healthy Weight Management:** Maintaining a healthy weight is essential for pelvic floor health. Excess weight can place added pressure on the pelvic floor muscles, contributing to urinary incontinence and pelvic organ prolapse.

6. **Protein Intake:** Adequate protein intake supports muscle health, including the pelvic floor muscles. Incorporating lean protein sources into your diet can

aid in muscle repair and maintenance.

Mind-Body Techniques:

1. **Mindfulness Meditation:** Mindfulness practices, including meditation and deep breathing, can help you connect with your body and improve awareness of the pelvic floor. This heightened awareness can aid in recognizing and addressing tension or dysfunction.

2. **Biofeedback:** Biofeedback techniques use electronic monitoring to provide real-time information about

muscle activity in the pelvic floor. This feedback can help you learn to control and relax these muscles effectively.

3. **Stress Reduction:** Chronic stress can contribute to pelvic floor tension and dysfunction. Stress reduction techniques, such as yoga, meditation, and progressive muscle relaxation, can alleviate tension and improve pelvic floor health.

4. **Pelvic Floor Physical Therapy:** Pelvic floor physical therapists are

trained to assess and treat pelvic floor issues. They may use techniques such as manual therapy, myofascial release, and biofeedback to address muscle imbalances and promote optimal pelvic floor function.

5. **Breathing Exercises:** Learning to coordinate your breath with pelvic floor muscle contractions can improve the effectiveness of Kegel exercises and enhance overall pelvic floor function.

6. **Pelvic Relaxation Techniques:** For individuals with pelvic pain

or hypertonic (overactive) pelvic floor muscles, relaxation techniques, such as guided imagery and progressive muscle relaxation, can be valuable in reducing muscle tension and discomfort.

7. **Seeking Professional Guidance:** If you're interested in incorporating mind-body techniques into your pelvic floor health routine, consider consulting a specialist in pelvic floor physical therapy or a mind-body therapist for personalized guidance.

By combining complementary exercises and stretches, dietary considerations, and mind-body techniques with your Kegel exercise routine, you can create a holistic approach to pelvic floor wellness. This comprehensive strategy can address various aspects of pelvic floor health, from muscle strength and flexibility to relaxation and overall well-being.

In the final chapter of this book, we will address common challenges and misconceptions related to Kegel exercises, provide tips for staying motivated, and offer answers to frequently asked questions to help you on your journey to optimal pelvic floor health.

CHAPTER 8

Common Challenges, Motivation, and FAQs

In this final chapter, we will address some common challenges people encounter when incorporating Kegel exercises into their routines. We'll also provide tips for staying motivated and answer frequently asked questions to ensure you have a successful and sustainable journey towards optimal pelvic floor health.

Common Challenges:

1. **Inconsistency:** One of the most common challenges is inconsistency in performing Kegel exercises. Life can get busy, and it's easy to forget or skip sessions. To overcome this, consider setting reminders on your phone or linking your Kegel routine to an existing daily habit, like brushing your teeth.

2. **Lack of Progress:** Some individuals may feel frustrated if they don't see immediate results. Remember that progress can be gradual, and it's essential

to be patient. Track your progress and celebrate small milestones to stay motivated.

3. **Difficulty Isolating Muscles:** Locating and isolating the pelvic floor muscles can be tricky, especially for beginners. If you're having trouble, don't hesitate to consult a pelvic floor physical therapist for guidance and feedback.

4. **Muscle Fatigue:** Overexerting the pelvic floor muscles can lead to fatigue or discomfort. It's crucial to find the right balance

between challenging your muscles and allowing them to recover. Avoid excessive repetitions or overly long contractions.

5. **Lack of Feedback:** Without professional guidance, it can be challenging to know if you're performing Kegel exercises correctly. Consider using biofeedback devices or seeking guidance from a pelvic floor physical therapist to ensure proper technique.

Staying Motivated:

1. **Set Clear Goals:** Establish specific, achievable goals for your Kegel exercise routine. Having a clear sense of purpose can motivate you to stay consistent.

2. **Create a Routine:** Incorporate Kegel exercises into your daily schedule. Treat them like any other appointment or commitment to increase the likelihood of sticking with them.

3. **Track Your Progress:** Keep a journal or use a Kegel exercise app to track your sessions and note any improvements in strength or

symptom relief. Progress tracking can be highly motivating.

4. **Join a Support Group:** Connecting with others who are on a similar journey can provide valuable support and motivation. Online forums, local support groups, or classes focused on pelvic floor health can be excellent resources.

5. **Reward Yourself:** Celebrate your successes along the way. Reward yourself when you achieve your goals or reach

milestones in your Kegel exercise routine.

6. **Mindfulness and Visualization:** Incorporate mindfulness techniques and visualization into your routine. By connecting with your body and visualizing the benefits of strong pelvic floor muscles, you can enhance your motivation.

Frequently Asked Questions (FAQs):

1. **How long does it take to see results from Kegel exercises?**

The timeline for results varies from person to person. Some individuals may notice improvements in a few weeks, while others may take several months. Consistency and patience are key.

2. Can I overdo Kegel exercises?

Yes, it's possible to overexert the pelvic floor muscles, leading to fatigue or discomfort. It's essential to find a balance between challenging your muscles and allowing them to recover. Avoid excessive repetitions or overly long contractions.

3. Are Kegel exercises suitable for everyone?

While Kegel exercises are generally beneficial, they may not be appropriate for everyone. It's essential to consult with a healthcare provider, especially if you have specific medical conditions or concerns. They can help you determine if Kegel exercises are right for you and provide guidance on the most suitable approach.

4. **Can I do Kegel exercises during pregnancy?**

Yes, Kegel exercises can be beneficial during pregnancy, as they can help prepare the pelvic floor muscles for labor and delivery. However, it's essential to consult with a healthcare provider to ensure you're performing them correctly and safely.

5. **What if I can't isolate the pelvic floor muscles?**

If you have difficulty isolating the pelvic floor muscles, consider seeking guidance from a pelvic floor physical therapist. They can provide personalized instruction and feedback to help you perform Kegel exercises correctly.

6. **Are there any side effects of Kegel exercises?**

When done correctly, Kegel exercises typically do not have significant side effects. However, overexertion or incorrect technique can lead to muscle fatigue or discomfort. If you experience any unusual symptoms, consult with a healthcare provider.

7. **Can men benefit from Kegel exercises?**

Yes, Kegel exercises can benefit men by improving urinary control, addressing erectile dysfunction, and enhancing ejaculatory control. Men with specific concerns should consult a healthcare provider for guidance.

8. **Is it possible to use Kegel exercises to treat pelvic floor disorders?**

In some cases, Kegel exercises may be part of the treatment plan for pelvic floor disorders. However, the approach varies depending on the specific condition and should be determined by a healthcare provider.

CONCLUSION

In closing, this chapter has addressed common challenges individuals may face when incorporating Kegel exercises into their routines, provided motivation strategies, and answered frequently asked questions. By staying committed to your pelvic floor health journey, seeking professional guidance when needed, and maintaining a balanced approach, you can achieve optimal pelvic floor wellness and enjoy the associated benefits for your overall well-being.

: Nurturing Your Pelvic Floor Health

In the pages of this book, we've embarked on a journey through the intricate world of pelvic floor health and explored the transformative power of Kegel exercises. From understanding the fundamentals of these exercises to tailoring them to specific populations, from embracing complementary practices to conquering common challenges, you've gained a comprehensive understanding of how to nurture your pelvic floor health.

Your pelvic floor is an intricate network of muscles and tissues, often overlooked until issues arise. But armed with knowledge, dedication, and a commitment to your well-being, you can take control of this vital part of your body.

Remember that optimal pelvic floor health extends beyond physical strength. It encompasses the holistic well-being of your body and mind. Your pelvic floor is not just a set of muscles; it's a cornerstone of your overall health, influencing everything from bladder control and sexual function to core stability and emotional well-being.

As you embark on your journey to nurturing your pelvic floor health, keep in mind the following key takeaways:

1. **Awareness is the First Step:** Recognizing the signs and symptoms of pelvic floor dysfunction is crucial. Early detection and seeking professional guidance are essential for effective management.

2. **Kegel Exercises are a Foundation:** Kegel exercises, named after Dr.

Arnold Kegel, are a powerful tool in strengthening and maintaining pelvic floor health. Proper technique, consistency, and patience are the keys to success.

3. **Tailoring Your Approach:** Kegel exercises can be adapted to meet the unique needs of different populations, including pregnant individuals, those in postpartum recovery, men seeking sexual health improvements, and aging adults.

4. **Complementary Practices Matter:**

Complementary exercises, stretches, dietary considerations, and mind-body techniques can enhance your pelvic floor health journey. These practices offer a holistic approach to wellness.

5. **Stay Committed and Motivated:** Challenges may arise, but maintaining consistency, setting clear goals, tracking progress, and seeking support from peers can help you stay motivated and dedicated to your pelvic floor health.

6. **Seek Professional Guidance:** If you have specific medical conditions or concerns, consulting with a healthcare provider, such as a pelvic floor physical therapist or urologist, is crucial. They can provide personalized guidance and ensure your safety and success.

Your pelvic floor health is a lifelong journey, and it's never too late to start. By embracing the knowledge and tools shared in this book, you've taken a significant step toward achieving and maintaining optimal pelvic floor wellness.

As you continue your path toward pelvic floor health, remember that it's not just about physical strength; it's about reclaiming control, restoring confidence, and nurturing your overall well-being. Your pelvic floor deserves your attention, care, and commitment, and the rewards of a healthy pelvic floor extend far beyond the physical. They touch every aspect of your life, enhancing your quality of life and allowing you to thrive.

With each Kegel exercise, each moment of mindfulness, and each step forward, you are investing in your own wellness. Your pelvic floor is your foundation, and by nurturing it, you are building a strong and resilient future for yourself.

So, here's to your pelvic floor health, to your well-being, and to a life lived to the fullest. May you walk this path with confidence, resilience, and the knowledge that you are in control of your pelvic floor health journey.